THE NEW MITOCHONDRIA DIET

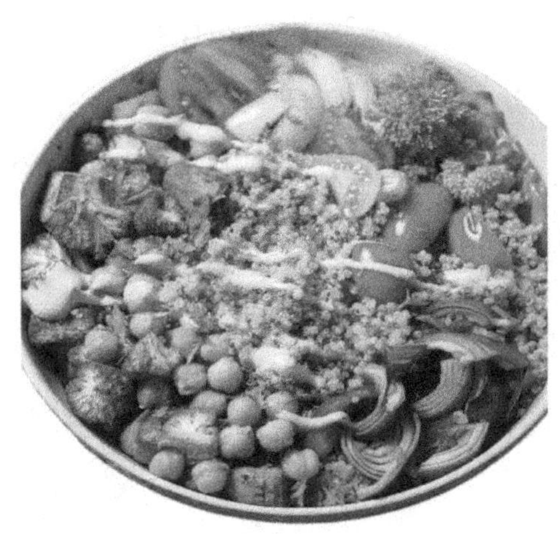

Nutrition Recipes to Manage Mitochondrial Dysfunction with 14 Days Meal Plan and Exercise

By

Dr. Clara Ramsey

Table of Contents

9 | The New Mitochondria Diet

Introduction

Imagine having tiny power plants in every cell of your body, each working tirelessly to generate the energy you need for nearly every action and function. These microscopic energy factories are called mitochondria, and they're not just essential—they're fundamental to life itself. Known as the "powerhouses of the cell," mitochondria produce more than 90% of the energy required by our organs to function optimally. From fueling muscle contractions to powering brain activity, mitochondria are the unseen heroes behind our vitality, stamina, and even mood stability.

My journey to writing The Complete Mitochondria Health Cookbook began with a simple question:

"What if our diet could directly influence the efficiency of these powerhouses?"

When I learned that nutrient-rich, antioxidant-filled foods can help protect and even strengthen mitochondrial function, I knew this book had the potential to be transformative for anyone looking to increase their energy, mental clarity, and resilience to stress.

In this cookbook, you'll not only discover recipes that nurture your mitochondria but also gain insights into which foods act as mitochondrial superstars. With each chapter, you'll learn how to take better care of these incredible cellular powerhouses, empowering you to feel more energized and healthy from the inside out.

Let's dive into the delicious world of mitochondria-friendly eating and unlock a new level of health and energy together!

Why Mitochondria Matter

Mitochondria are often referred to as the "powerhouses of the cell," and for a good reason—they generate the energy necessary for nearly every cellular function in our bodies.

These tiny, bean-shaped structures convert nutrients into adenosine triphosphate (ATP), the energy currency our cells use to perform countless vital tasks. They are not only essential for physical energy but are also critical for brain function, metabolic health, and immune responses.

Beyond energy production, mitochondria play a key role in cellular resilience and aging.

Healthy mitochondria are essential for supporting longevity, physical strength, cognitive clarity, and overall well-being. As we age, mitochondrial efficiency often declines, contributing to reduced energy levels, slower metabolism, and even cognitive impairment.

Moreover, emerging research links poor mitochondrial function to various health conditions, including neurodegenerative diseases, metabolic disorders, and cardiovascular diseases.

Supporting and strengthening our mitochondria is therefore essential for maintaining vitality and preventing chronic illnesses. The food we consume can significantly influence mitochondrial health—by either supporting energy production or causing oxidative stress that can damage these vital organelles.

How This Cookbook Supports Your Mitochondria

The New Mitochondria Cookbook is designed to empower you with the tools and recipes to enhance mitochondrial function through balanced, nutrient-dense meals. Here's how this cookbook supports your journey toward optimal mitochondrial health:

Focus on Key Nutrients for Mitochondrial Health

The recipes in this book are carefully curated to be rich in nutrients known to support mitochondrial function. Ingredients include foods high in antioxidants (to protect against oxidative damage), omega-3 fatty acids (for cell membrane support), and B vitamins (essential for energy production).

By incorporating these recipes into your daily routine, you're consistently providing your mitochondria with the nutrients they need to function optimally.

Antioxidant-Rich Recipes for Cellular Defense

Mitochondria are especially vulnerable to oxidative stress, a process in which free radicals damage cellular structures, leading to inflammation and impaired function. Antioxidants from fruits, vegetables, and spices like turmeric and ginger play a vital role in neutralizing these free radicals.

This cookbook includes antioxidant-rich dishes designed to protect your mitochondria from oxidative stress, supporting longevity and reducing cellular aging.

Protein for Repair and Maintenance

Mitochondria rely on proteins for energy production and cellular repair. The book includes recipes with high-quality protein sources, from plant-based options like lentils and quinoa to lean animal sources, catering to different dietary preferences.

These recipes help ensure you get enough amino acids to maintain mitochondrial efficiency and cellular health.

Energy-Boosting Carbohydrates

While a low-carbohydrate diet has its benefits, glucose is still a crucial fuel for mitochondrial energy production. The recipes in this cookbook include complex carbohydrates from sources like whole grains, sweet potatoes, and legumes, providing a steady supply of glucose without spiking blood sugar.

These slow-burning carbohydrates support sustained energy levels throughout the day, enhancing mitochondrial endurance.

Meal Planning for Consistency

One of the most effective ways to support mitochondrial health is through consistent, balanced eating. This cookbook offers meal planning tips and guides, making it easier to incorporate a mitochondrial-supportive diet into your daily life.

By following these meal plans, you create a sustainable approach to nourishing your mitochondria, ensuring long-term benefits for energy, vitality, and resilience.

Mitochondria are the unsung heroes of cellular health, and this cookbook is your guide to keeping them robust and resilient. With each recipe, you're taking a step toward a lifestyle that values and prioritizes mitochondrial wellness, ultimately supporting your body's natural ability to generate energy and maintain vitality at any age.

By feeding your cells well, you're not just cooking for taste—you're cooking for life, longevity, and lasting health.

Chapter One

Understanding Mitochondrial Health

What Are Mitochondria?

When you hear the word "mitochondria," you might flash back to a high school biology class where they were described as the "powerhouses of the cell." While that's a true, it's a simplification of what mitochondria really are and why they're vital to our health.

Think of them as the miniature engines within each of your cells, tirelessly working to fuel everything you do—from movin g your muscles to even thinking and feeling. If mitochondria are compromised, energy dwindles, and our bodies begin to feel it, often in ways we don't immediately understand.

The Mighty Mitochondria

Mitochondria generate energy by converting the food we eat and the oxygen we breathe into ATP (adenosine triphosphate), the chemical fuel for all cellular activities. This isn't just important for athletes or people with physically demanding jobs—it's essential for every one of us, as ATP powers almost every process in the body.

Imagine mitochondria as tiny engines in each cell, humming quietly and efficiently in the background. But just like a car engine, they need the right fuel and care to keep running smoothly.

If mitochondria are neglected or damaged, energy production drops.

The results? Fatigue, cognitive fog, slowed metabolism, and even accelerated aging.

I remember when I first felt that symptoms—tiredness that just didn't seem to go away, even after a good night's sleep.

After researching and learning more, I realized that what I was feeling might actually be linked to my mitochondria, and so I set out on a journey to boost their health.

Why Mitochondria Matter for Wellness and Longevity

Mitochondria are not only about energy. They are essential for managing and regulating cell health, from repairing damage to managing apoptosis, the natural process of cell death.

Keeping these cellular powerhouses strong is one of the keys to living a vibrant, active, and resilient life. Poor mitochondrial health has been linked to many chronic diseases, including neurodegenerative conditions like Alzheimer's, metabolic syndromes like diabetes, and cardiovascular diseases.

This topic became real to me when a close friend was diagnosed with a mitochondrial disorder—a reminder that mitochondrial health is crucial for everyone, not just those dealing with illness. Supporting mitochondrial health helps protect us from many of the ailments that may otherwise impair our quality of life as we age.

What Affects Mitochondrial Health?

The lifestyle we lead has a profound effect on mitochondrial health. Chronic stress, a high-sugar diet, lack of physical activity, exposure to toxins, and even certain medications can all weaken these vital structures. For instance, diets that are high in processed sugars can cause "oxidative stress," a process that produces free radicals and damages cell components, including mitochondria.

On the other hand, eating a balanced diet, staying active, and managing stress levels can keep our mitochondria functioning optimally.

I used to rely on sugar-filled snacks for energy during busy days. But once I realized the impact this could have on my mitochondria, I started making small but meaningful changes—like switching to whole foods and prioritizing protein and complex carbohydrates. Within weeks, I noticed an improvement in my energy levels and overall sense of well-being.

Supporting Your Mitochondria Through Diet

This cookbook is designed to help you support your mitochondria through thoughtful, nutrient-rich recipes. Foods rich in antioxidants (like berries and leafy greens), healthy fats (such as avocado and nuts), and proteins all play a crucial role in nourishing these tiny engines. The recipes in this book incorporate these ingredients in creative, delicious ways, making it easier to adopt a mitochondrial-friendly diet without feeling deprived.

Each meal you prepare from this cookbook is a step toward healthier, more resilient mitochondria, supporting energy production, mental clarity, and longevity. Cooking with a focus on mitochondrial health isn't just about adding years to your life—it's about enhancing the quality of those years, so you can enjoy the energy to do what you love and live fully.

The Vital Role of Mitochondria in Energy Production

When we consume food, mitochondria are where the real magic happens. They take oxygen and nutrients from our meals and transform them into ATP through a process called cellular respiration. This process involves a complex sequence of biochemical reactions—kind of like a well-orchestrated assembly line—that converts fuel into energy. ATP is then transported throughout the cell to power everything from muscle contractions to brain functions.

Think about those times you've felt sluggish, even after a good night's sleep or a healthy meal. Often, it's because your mitochondria aren't working as efficiently as they should.

In my experience, I started noticing this when I was overwhelmed with work and surviving on caffeine and processed snacks.

The constant fatigue wasn't just from a lack of sleep; my mitochondria weren't getting the nutrients they needed to function optimally. It was like trying to run a car on low-quality fuel.

When mitochondria function well, we feel energized and resilient. However, when they become damaged due to stress, poor diet, lack of exercise, or exposure to toxins, our energy levels drop. Damaged mitochondria also produce more free radicals, which can lead to oxidative stress and further harm cells. Over time, this can contribute to aging and even chronic illnesses.

How This Relates to Our Everyday Lives

In practical terms, supporting mitochondrial health means embracing lifestyle choices that promote optimal energy production and resilience. Proper nutrition, regular physical activity, stress management, and enough sleep are key factors. It's like maintaining a car with regular check-ups, quality fuel, and occasional breaks—it makes a noticeable difference in performance.

By understanding how mitochondria work, we gain a new perspective on our health. This is why this cookbook is so special: each recipe is carefully crafted to provide the nutrients that nourish these tiny but mighty structures. Whether you're adding more antioxidant-rich foods to combat free radicals or including healthy fats that support mitochondrial membranes, each meal becomes a step toward fueling your body's natural powerhouse.

Chapter Two

Identifying Mitochondrial Needs

When we think about health and energy, it's easy to focus on what's happening on the surface—how we feel, how active we are, or how we're sleeping. But the real "core" of our energy lies in the mitochondria, the tiny structures within cells that convert nutrients into power.

Each of us has individual mitochondrial needs, influenced by lifestyle, diet, stress, and even genetics. Knowing what our mitochondria require can feel like unlocking a new layer of wellness, helping us understand why we feel energized some days and sluggish on others.

Personally, I remember experiencing afternoon slumps that no amount of coffee could fix. It felt like my body was constantly running low on fuel, despite my best efforts to eat "healthy." But when I learned more about mitochondria and their specific nutrient needs, it changed my approach to eating and living.

I realized that simple adjustments, like including foods high in antioxidants or incorporating regular movement, had a noticeable effect on my energy levels.

Key Nutrients for Mitochondrial Function

Mitochondria rely on a range of nutrients to keep them running smoothly. Each nutrient has a specific role in energy production, from supporting the cellular processes of ATP production to repairing damage caused by free radicals.

Here are some of the essential nutrients and why they matter:

Coenzyme Q10 (CoQ10): Often called the "spark plug" for mitochondria, CoQ10 is essential for ATP production. It helps shuttle electrons within the mitochondria, a key step in energy conversion. Without enough CoQ10, mitochondria struggle to produce energy efficiently, which can lead to fatigue.

For example, I noticed a real difference when I added CoQ10-rich foods like spinach and cauliflower into my meals. It felt like an added layer of natural energy.

B Vitamins (especially B2, B3, B5, B6, and B12): B vitamins are involved in multiple steps of the mitochondrial energy cycle. They help convert nutrients into usable energy, and deficiencies can often lead to low energy and even mood fluctuations.

For instance, B12 and folate are critical for cellular function and repair. When I started including more B-rich foods like whole grains and leafy greens, I noticed improved mental clarity and a sense of steadiness throughout the day.

Magnesium: This mineral is often underrated in mitochondrial health, but it plays a critical role in over 300 enzymatic reactions in the body, including ATP production.

Magnesium is also essential for maintaining mitochondrial integrity and reducing oxidative stress. Foods like pumpkin seeds, almonds, and dark chocolate offer good magnesium sources and have become my go-to snacks to keep my energy stable.

Antioxidants (Vitamin C, Vitamin E, and Selenium): Mitochondria naturally produce free radicals during energy production, but without enough antioxidants, these free radicals can cause damage. Antioxidants like vitamin C, vitamin E, and selenium help neutralize these harmful molecules.

I love adding bright-colored fruits and vegetables like berries, citrus, and tomatoes to my diet for an antioxidant boost.

Healthy Fats (Omega-3s): Omega-3 fatty acids help maintain mitochondrial membrane health, which is crucial for optimal function. These fats act like a flexible, protective layer around the mitochondria, supporting their structure and function.

Walnuts, flaxseeds, and olive oil are great sources of omega-3s, and I incorporate them into my daily diet for both brain and energy benefits.

Identifying what your mitochondria need can feel empowering, and it doesn't require an overhaul of your entire lifestyle. Small changes—like focusing on nutrient-dense foods, staying hydrated, and prioritizing sleep—can make a noticeable difference.

For example, swapping processed snacks for a handful of almonds or adding a serving of leafy greens to your meals can help fuel your mitochondria.

In my journey, I found that the more I honored my mitochondria with the nutrients they need, the more I noticed lasting energy and fewer "crash" moments throughout the day.

This is what this cookbook is all about: helping you create meals that don't just taste great but also support your cellular health from within. Each recipe is crafted with these mitochondrial needs in mind, offering a delicious way to give your body's powerhouses the fuel they crave.

Embracing this mitochondrial approach to eating transforms every meal into a step toward sustained energy, better mood, and vibrant health.

Signs of Mitochondrial Dysfunction

Mitochondrial dysfunction can be subtle, often manifesting in ways that are easily mistaken for everyday fatigue or stress.

Since mitochondria are our cellular powerhouses, any disruption in their function can affect every part of the body, leading to a range of symptoms that impact physical, mental, and even emotional well-being.

When I first experienced what I now recognize as symptoms of mitochondrial dysfunction, I attributed my constant tiredness to a busy schedule. But as the symptoms persisted, I began to see patterns beyond just being "run-down."

Here are some common signs of mitochondrial dysfunction, along with personal experience that may resonate with anyone struggling to maintain their energy levels.

1. Persistent Fatigue

Fatigue is often one of the earliest and most noticeable symptoms. Unlike typical tiredness, this fatigue doesn't improve with rest and may feel like a pervasive lack of energy. When your cells aren't producing enough ATP (the energy currency of the body), even simple tasks can feel exhausting.

I remember needing a nap after activities that wouldn't normally tire me out, like grocery shopping or a walk around the block. It was as if my "battery" was constantly half-full, no matter how much sleep or relaxation I got.

2. Muscle Weakness and Pain

Mitochondria are critical for muscle function because they provide the energy muscles need to contract and move. Muscle weakness, cramping, or even unexplained pain can signal that something isn't right at the cellular level.

Personally, I experienced unusual soreness after moderate workouts, which I initially brushed off as "just getting older." But when I felt pain even after gentle stretches, I began to suspect that something deeper was at play.

3. Brain Fog and Memory Problems

Mental clarity and memory are deeply connected to mitochondrial function, as the brain is a highly energy-demanding organ. When mitochondria struggle, cognitive issues like brain fog, forgetfulness, and difficulty concentrating often arise.

I remember sitting down to work, only to find myself re-reading the same paragraph multiple times because I couldn't retain the information. It was frustrating and made me feel as if I was in a constant mental fog.

4. Poor Exercise Tolerance

Many people with mitochondrial dysfunction notice that they can't tolerate exercise as they once did. Activities like running or even brisk walking become challenging, with prolonged recovery times after exertion.

For me, I realized something was wrong when I could barely finish my usual bike ride without needing multiple breaks. My muscles felt heavy and uncooperative, signaling that my cells weren't producing the energy I needed.

5. Gastrointestinal Issues

Mitochondria are also vital for the smooth functioning of our digestive system, influencing gut motility and nutrient absorption. Symptoms like bloating, constipation, or even unexplained stomach pain can sometimes point to mitochondrial dysfunction.

I was surprised to learn that some of my occasional digestive discomfort was likely related to my cells' energy production issues. Understanding this connection has made it easier to manage my symptoms with diet and lifestyle changes.

6. Mood Changes

The brain's emotional regulation systems also rely on mitochondrial function, so mood changes such as increased anxiety, irritability, or depression can be another red flag.

For me, these changes crept in gradually. I noticed that I was feeling more overwhelmed and irritable in situations that previously wouldn't have affected me. Recognizing that my mitochondria played a role helped me address these mood changes with greater self-compassion.

Why Recognizing These Signs Matters

Mitochondrial dysfunction often masquerades as common issues we might overlook or attribute to stress, aging, or lifestyle. However, understanding these signs allows for early intervention, often through diet, exercise, and targeted nutrients that support mitochondrial health. By addressing the root of these symptoms, we can improve not only energy levels but also overall health and quality of life.

This is exactly why this cookbook was created. The recipes within are designed to support mitochondrial health, giving your cells the nutrients they need to power through each day with resilience and vitality.

Making even small, consistent changes in diet can have a profound impact, providing lasting energy, mental clarity, and an overall sense of well-being. This journey is not just about adding new foods to your plate; it's about empowering your body's powerhouses—your mitochondria—to thrive.

Chapter Two

Mitochondria-Supporting Foods and Top Antioxidant-Rich Ingredients

If you've ever found yourself feeling drained, sluggish, or mentally foggy, it could be that your mitochondria are in need of a little extra support. These tiny yet mighty powerhouses in each of our cells rely on nutrient-dense, antioxidant-rich foods to function at their best.

When our mitochondria have what they need, we feel energized, clear-minded, and more resilient. But without the right fuel, they (and we) start to run on empty. I personally noticed a difference once I began incorporating more mitochondria-boosting foods into my diet, feeling a steady increase in energy and mental clarity.

Here's a guide to some of the best foods and ingredients to support mitochondrial health, along with a closer look at the role antioxidants play in protecting and powering these cellular engines.

1. Leafy Greens: Spinach, Kale, and Swiss Chard

Leafy greens are rich in magnesium, a mineral crucial for ATP production in the mitochondria. When we eat greens, our cells get the "spark" they need to keep our energy levels up.

Adding a handful of spinach to a smoothie or enjoying a crisp kale salad with a sprinkle of lemon brings out the earthy, slightly sweet flavors that make these greens a joy to eat.

I found that adding greens to my diet even in small amounts, like a handful in my lunch, helped me avoid the midday energy dip.

2. Berries: Blueberries, Strawberries, and Raspberries

Berries are famous for their high antioxidant content, especially vitamin C and anthocyanins. Antioxidants are like a protective shield for our mitochondria, reducing oxidative stress that can damage cells.

When we enjoy a bowl of fresh berries or a berry-packed smoothie, the sweet, tangy flavors flood our taste buds and provide our mitochondria with a vibrant shield against free radicals.

Since incorporating berries, I've felt more refreshed and even noticed my skin looking healthier—a bonus from the high antioxidant intake.

3. Nuts and Seeds: Almonds, Walnuts, Chia, and Flax Seeds

Rich in healthy fats and antioxidants like vitamin E, nuts and seeds support mitochondrial function and protect cell membranes from damage. Nuts also provide essential fatty acids that are a key component of cell membranes. I like to add chia seeds to my yogurt or sprinkle some walnuts over my salad—the crunch and subtle flavors elevate each meal while nourishing my cells.

4. Fatty Fish: Salmon, Sardines, and Mackerel

Omega-3 fatty acids found in fatty fish, like salmon are crucial for mitochondrial health. These healthy fats support the structure and function of cell membranes, making it easier for mitochondria to produce energy.

The rich, savory flavor of a grilled salmon fillet is deeply satisfying, and knowing it's fueling my cells makes it even better. Eating fish just a few times a week made a noticeable difference in my stamina during busy days.

5. Citrus Fruits: Oranges, Lemons, and Grapefruits

Citrus fruits are excellent sources of vitamin C, a potent antioxidant that helps protect mitochondria from damage. The bright, refreshing taste of a glass of lemon water in the morning or an orange as a snack is not only uplifting but gives your mitochondria an extra layer of defense. Since adding citrus to my mornings, I feel more energized and alert.

6. Cruciferous Vegetables: Broccoli, Brussels Sprouts, and Cauliflower

Cruciferous vegetables contain compounds like sulforaphane that support mitochondrial function and encourage detoxification processes in the body.

These vegetables bring a wonderful earthy flavor to dishes and add a unique texture that can be enjoyed steamed, roasted, or raw. I've found that making a small bowl of roasted broccoli or Brussels sprouts as a side dish adds both nutrition and deliciousness to my meals.

7. Dark Chocolate: Choose High Cocoa Content (70% or More)

Good news for chocolate lovers! Dark chocolate, especially those with high cocoa content, contains antioxidants that benefit mitochondrial function and blood flow.

The rich, slightly bitter taste of dark chocolate can be incredibly satisfying as a treat, knowing it's also helping my cells. A small square of dark chocolate after lunch is my go-to treat that lifts my mood and gives my mitochondria some extra love.

8. Avocado: Packed with Healthy Fats and Fiber

Avocado is a nutritional powerhouse that provides monounsaturated fats, essential for maintaining mitochondrial health and supporting energy production. Its creamy texture and mild flavor pair well with so many dishes. Adding avocado to toast or a salad not only keeps me full but also fuels my cells for sustained energy.

9. Sweet Potatoes: A Great Source of Beta-Carotene and Fiber

Sweet potatoes are rich in beta-carotene, which supports cellular health and provides a steady release of energy. The sweet, comforting flavor of a baked sweet potato with a dash of cinnamon makes it a versatile ingredient that can be enjoyed in both sweet and savory dishes. I find that sweet potatoes help me feel energized and grounded throughout the day.

10. Herbs and Spices: Turmeric, Ginger, and Garlic

Turmeric, ginger, and garlic have natural anti-inflammatory and antioxidant properties that help protect mitochondria. These spices add warmth and depth to dishes, from curries to teas, and they come with a host of benefits. Adding a pinch of turmeric to my meals has become a daily ritual for me, knowing it's not only adding flavor but also supporting my cells.

Why Antioxidants Are Key to Mitochondrial Health

Antioxidants are crucial because they neutralize free radicals—unstable molecules that can damage cells, including mitochondria. Our cells naturally produce free radicals, but when their levels rise due to stress, pollution, or poor diet, they can outpace our body's antioxidant defenses, leading to oxidative stress and, ultimately, mitochondrial damage. This damage contributes to aging, fatigue, and a host of other health issues.

Incorporating antioxidant-rich foods like berries, leafy greens, and dark chocolate helps balance this oxidative load. These foods serve as our mitochondria's armor, allowing them to work efficiently and provide the energy we need. I've found that simply adding a few of these antioxidant-rich foods each day has a noticeable impact, helping me feel more resilient and energetic.

By including these mitochondria-supporting foods in your daily diet, you're not just eating to fuel your body—you're also taking proactive steps to protect your cells and support long-term health. Each meal can be an opportunity to give your body the tools it needs to thrive. This approach has not only changed how I feel but also how I think about food and self-care. Remember, small changes lead to big results over time. So, enjoy these foods, knowing they're helping you thrive from the cellular level up.

Foods to Avoid for Optimal Mitochondrial Health

When it comes to supporting our mitochondria, what we don't eat can be as important as what we do. Just as certain foods can give our cells the energy and resilience they need, others can slow down or even damage these crucial powerhouses. It's a balance I learned firsthand after noticing my own energy levels fluctuating wildly; cutting back on certain foods really made a difference.

Let's dive into which foods can interfere with mitochondrial health and why they're best kept to a minimum.

1. Processed Foods and Refined Sugars

Processed foods and refined sugars are everywhere—from fast foods to packaged snacks—and though they're convenient, they can be a big burden on our mitochondria. High in empty calories, added sugars, and unhealthy fats, processed foods offer little nutritional value but a lot of oxidative stress.

Sugar, in particular, causes insulin spikes that can contribute to inflammation, which is tough on mitochondria. I used to crave sugary snacks in the afternoon, but switching to a handful of berries gave me a more even energy boost without the crash.

Tip: When you crave something sweet, try fresh fruit or a small piece of dark chocolate (70% or higher cocoa). The natural sugars are gentler on your system, and the antioxidants in dark chocolate even help protect your cells.

2. Trans Fats and Hydrogenated Oils

Trans fats, often found in margarine, shortening, and many processed baked goods, are a true enemy of mitochondrial health. These fats interfere with the cell's lipid membranes, making it harder for mitochondria to function and for cells to communicate properly.

For a long time, I didn't think much about which oils were used in my food until I learned how much impact it could have on my energy. Switching from fried, oily foods to grilled or baked options gave me a noticeable boost in vitality.

Tip: Use olive oil, avocado oil, or coconut oil when cooking at home. These fats provide healthy fuel and are much easier on the mitochondria than processed oils.

3. Artificial Sweeteners and Additives

While cutting sugar is a smart move for mitochondrial health, replacing it with artificial sweeteners like aspartame or saccharin isn't the solution. These additives can disrupt gut health, causing an imbalance in gut bacteria that influences mitochondrial function.

After trying "sugar-free" sodas and snacks, I found that these alternatives didn't give me the energy boost I hoped for; instead, they left me feeling tired and bloated.

Tip: If you're looking for a sugar substitute, try natural options like stevia or monk fruit in moderation. They add sweetness without adding stress to your cells.

4. Alcohol

Alcohol is one of the quickest ways to drain mitochondrial energy. When we drink, our body has to work overtime to process the alcohol, which takes up resources our mitochondria could otherwise use for energy production. On top of that, alcohol leads to oxidative stress and can damage mitochondrial DNA over time.

After social gatherings, I would often feel completely drained; it turned out that even a little alcohol was enough to throw off my energy levels the next day.

Tip: If you enjoy a drink now and then, opt for antioxidant-rich red wine in moderation. Or, try sparkling water with a twist of lemon—it's refreshing, and your mitochondria will thank you.

5. High-Sodium Foods

Foods high in sodium, like canned soups, chips, and fast foods, can cause inflammation and oxidative stress in the body, which can affect mitochondria over time. I found that cutting back on salty snacks and processed foods helped me feel less bloated and more energetic throughout the day.

Tip: Flavor your food with herbs and spices instead of salt. Not only do these add depth to your meals, but many spices like turmeric and ginger also have antioxidant properties that support mitochondria.

6. Red and Processed Meats

Red meat and processed meats, like hot dogs and sausages, can be difficult for our bodies to break down and metabolize. This can lead to a buildup of byproducts that create oxidative stress and inflammation.

For a while, I was in the habit of grabbing quick processed meats for lunch, but shifting to more plant-based options made a difference in how light and energetic I felt post-meal.

Tip: Substitute red meat with fish or plant-based proteins a few times a week. When you do enjoy red meat, opt for lean, grass-fed options, which are healthier for you and easier on your cells.

7. Excess Caffeine

While moderate caffeine can have some benefits, too much of it can backfire. Excessive caffeine stimulates the central nervous system, which can make you feel jittery and anxious, increasing stress hormones that challenge mitochondrial health. I used to rely on coffee for energy throughout the day, but now I limit myself to one cup in the morning. It's amazing how much steadier my energy feels without the afternoon caffeine crashes.

Tip: If you're looking for a gentler energy boost, try green tea or matcha. Both contain antioxidants and provide a smoother, more sustained lift than coffee.

Why Avoiding These Foods Makes a Difference

It's easy to underestimate how much our everyday food choices impact mitochondrial health. Each small choice—whether it's picking whole foods over processed ones, or swapping high-sugar snacks for fresh fruit—contributes to building a supportive environment for these vital cell structures.

By giving our mitochondria the fuel they need and cutting back on foods that cause strain, we're essentially investing in better energy, mental clarity, and overall resilience.

Since making these changes, I've felt a profound improvement in how I feel day-to-day, with fewer dips in energy and a greater sense of wellbeing. It's a reminder that even the smallest adjustments to our diet can lead to big rewards in health and vitality.

Chapter Three

Breakfast Recipes For Mitochondrial Health

Here's a selection of breakfast recipes tailored for mitochondrial health. These recipes are rich in antioxidants, fiber, healthy fats, and essential nutrients to support energy production at the cellular level. They incorporate ingredients that boost mitochondrial function and maintain balanced energy throughout the day.

Berry Chia Pudding

A Creamy, cool, and slightly sweet with a hint of vanilla, bursting with the tartness of fresh berries.

Ingredients

2 tbsp chia seeds

1 cup almond or coconut milk

1/2 tsp vanilla extract

1/4 cup mixed berries (blueberries, strawberries, raspberries)

1 tsp honey or maple syrup (optional)

Instructions

In a small bowl, mix chia seeds with almond milk and vanilla. Stir well.

Cover and refrigerate overnight or at least 4 hours until it thickens to a pudding-like consistency.

Top with fresh berries and a drizzle of honey or maple syrup if desired.

Health Benefits: Chia seeds are rich in omega-3s and fiber, supporting brain health and mitochondrial function. Berries are packed with antioxidants, which protect mitochondria from oxidative stress.

Avocado & Spinach Smoothie

A Smooth and creamy with a refreshing green taste and a hint of sweetness.

Ingredients

1/2 ripe avocado

1 cup spinach

1/2 banana

1 tbsp chia or flax seeds

1 cup coconut water or almond milk

Instructions

Combine all ingredients in a blender.

Blend until smooth and creamy.

Pour into a glass and enjoy immediately.

Health Benefits: Avocado provides healthy fats that fuel mitochondria, and spinach is rich in magnesium and iron, which are crucial for energy production.

Quinoa Breakfast Bowl with Berries and Almonds

Nutty, warm, and slightly sweet, complemented by the crunch of almonds and the freshness of berries.

Ingredients

1/2 cup cooked quinoa

1/4 cup mixed berries

1 tbsp chopped almonds

1 tsp honey or maple syrup

1/2 tsp cinnamon

Instructions

In a bowl, combine cooked quinoa with cinnamon and honey.

Top with berries and almonds for added crunch and flavor.

Serve warm or at room temperature.

Health Benefits: Quinoa is a complete protein that aids in cellular repair. Berries provide antioxidants, while almonds supply healthy fats to support mitochondrial energy production.

Sweet Potato & Kale Hash

Warm and earthy with a slight sweetness from sweet potatoes and a savory kick from kale.

Ingredients

1 small sweet potato, diced

1 cup kale, chopped

1 tbsp olive oil

Salt and pepper to taste

1/4 tsp paprika (optional)

Instructions

Heat olive oil in a pan over medium heat.

Add diced sweet potato and cook for 5–7 minutes until slightly tender.

Add chopped kale and season with salt, pepper, and paprika.

Cook for another 5 minutes until kale is wilted and sweet potatoes are fully cooked.

Health Benefits: Sweet potatoes are rich in antioxidants and complex carbs for sustained energy, while kale is a powerhouse of vitamins supporting mitochondrial health.

Greek Yogurt with Walnuts & Honey

Creamy and rich with a hint of sweetness from honey and crunch from walnuts.

Ingredients

1 cup Greek yogurt

1 tbsp chopped walnuts

1 tsp honey

1/4 tsp cinnamon (optional)

Instructions

Scoop Greek yogurt into a bowl.

Top with walnuts, honey, and a sprinkle of cinnamon if desired.

Health Benefits: Greek yogurt provides probiotics for gut health, essential for nutrient absorption, while walnuts offer healthy fats and antioxidants that protect mitochondria.

Spinach & Mushroom Scramble

Savory, soft, and earthy with a mild garlic aroma.

Ingredients

2 eggs (or egg substitute)

1/2 cup spinach, chopped

1/4 cup mushrooms, sliced

1 tsp olive oil

Salt and pepper to taste

Instructions

Heat olive oil in a pan over medium heat, then add mushrooms and cook until tender.

Add spinach and cook until wilted.

Pour in eggs, season with salt and pepper, and scramble until fully cooked.

Health Benefits: Eggs contain B vitamins, essential for mitochondrial energy production, and spinach provides magnesium, which is crucial for ATP synthesis.

Almond Butter & Banana Toast

Creamy and nutty with the natural sweetness of banana.

Ingredients

1 slice whole-grain bread

1 tbsp almond butter

1/2 banana, sliced

1/4 tsp chia seeds (optional)

Instructions

Toast the bread to desired crispness.

Spread almond butter on top and layer with banana slices.

Sprinkle with chia seeds for extra crunch.

Health Benefits: Whole grains and bananas provide steady energy, while almond butter contains healthy fats and protein that fuel mitochondria.

Coconut & Berry Smoothie Bowl

Thick, fruity, and refreshing with a creamy coconut taste.

Ingredients

1/2 cup coconut milk

1/2 cup frozen berries

1/4 cup spinach

1 tbsp chia seeds

Instructions

Blend all ingredients until thick and smooth.

Pour into a bowl and top with fresh berries or coconut flakes.

Health Benefits: Coconut provides MCTs (medium-chain triglycerides) for quick energy, while berries offer antioxidants to protect mitochondrial health.

Oatmeal with Chia and Blueberries

Creamy and warm with bursts of berry flavor and a touch of nutty chia crunch.

Ingredients

1/2 cup oats

1 cup water or almond milk

1 tbsp chia seeds

1/4 cup blueberries

1 tsp honey or maple syrup (optional)

Instructions

In a saucepan, bring water or almond milk to a boil, add oats and cook until thickened.

Stir in chia seeds and top with blueberries and honey.

Health Benefits: Oats provide fiber and steady-release energy, while chia seeds are rich in omega-3s that benefit mitochondrial health.

Apple & Almond Butter Roll-Ups

Crisp and sweet with a creamy, nutty filling.

Ingredients

1 apple, sliced

1 tbsp almond butter

1/4 tsp cinnamon (optional)

Instructions

Spread a small amount of almond butter on each apple slice.

Sprinkle with cinnamon for extra flavor.

Health Benefits: Apples are rich in antioxidants, and almond butter provides protein and healthy fats, both of which support mitochondrial health.

Each of these breakfasts helps energize your day and provides the nutrients that fuel your cells' powerhouses, setting a foundation for sustained vitality.

Lunch Recipes For Mitochondrial Health

Here are nutrient-packed, sustained-energy lunch recipes that cater to mitochondrial health. Each recipe is crafted with ingredients known to support mitochondrial function, ensuring steady energy and essential nutrients to keep your cells performing at their best.

Quinoa and Roasted Veggie Bowl

Warm and hearty, with a nutty, slightly sweet aroma and a satisfying mix of textures from tender roasted vegetables and fluffy quinoa.

Ingredients

1 cup cooked quinoa

1/2 cup broccoli florets

1/2 cup cubed sweet potato

1/4 red onion, sliced

1 tbsp olive oil

Salt and pepper to taste

1 tbsp tahini

1 tsp lemon juice

Instructions

Preheat oven to 400°F (200°C). Toss broccoli, sweet potato, and onion with olive oil, salt, and pepper.

Roast on a baking sheet for 20-25 minutes until tender.

Combine quinoa and roasted veggies in a bowl. Drizzle with tahini and lemon juice.

Health Benefits: Quinoa is rich in protein and fiber, promoting satiety and steady energy. Sweet potatoes add complex carbs and beta-carotene for antioxidant support.

Avocado Chickpea Wrap

Creamy and satisfying with a hint of spice, combining smooth avocado and mashed chickpeas in a wrap that's easy to enjoy on the go.

Ingredients

1 whole-wheat tortilla

1/2 avocado, mashed

1/2 cup chickpeas, mashed

1 tbsp lemon juice

Salt, pepper, and a pinch of chili flakes

Handful of spinach leaves

Instructions

Mix avocado, chickpeas, lemon juice, salt, pepper, and chili flakes in a bowl.

Spread mixture on a tortilla and layer with spinach leaves.

Roll up the wrap and slice in half.

Health Benefits: Avocado offers healthy fats essential for energy metabolism, while chickpeas provide fiber and protein for prolonged satiety.

Kale and Black Bean Salad with Lime Dressing

Crisp and tangy with earthy flavors and a zesty lime aroma.

Ingredients

2 cups kale, chopped

1/2 cup black beans, drained and rinsed

1/4 cup diced bell pepper

1/4 cup shredded carrots

1 tbsp olive oil

Juice of 1 lime

Salt and pepper to taste

Instructions

Massage chopped kale with a little salt to soften.

Add black beans, bell pepper, and carrots.

Drizzle with olive oil and lime juice, tossing to coat.

Health Benefits: Kale is a superfood rich in antioxidants, while black beans offer protein and fiber for blood sugar stability.

Spinach and Sweet Potato Frittata

Savory and fluffy with a hint of sweetness from roasted sweet potato, perfect for a warm, comforting lunch.

Ingredients

1 small sweet potato, diced

1 cup spinach, chopped

3 eggs

Salt and pepper to taste

1 tsp olive oil

Instructions

Sauté diced sweet potato in olive oil over medium heat until soft.

Add spinach and cook until wilted.

Whisk eggs with salt and pepper, pour over veggies, and cook until set.

Health Benefits: Eggs provide high-quality protein, and sweet potatoes are a great source of complex carbohydrates.

Lentil and Veggie Stuffed Peppers

Soft, savory peppers filled with flavorful lentils and veggies, with a hint of spice.

Ingredients

2 bell peppers, halved and seeded

1/2 cup cooked lentils

1/4 cup diced tomatoes

1/4 cup chopped zucchini

Salt, pepper, and Italian herbs

Instructions

Preheat oven to 375°F (190°C). Mix lentils, tomatoes, zucchini, salt, pepper, and herbs.

Fill pepper halves with mixture and bake for 20-25 minutes.

Health Benefits: Lentils are packed with protein and iron, promoting energy and immune support.

Zucchini Noodles with Pesto and Cherry Tomatoes

Fresh and vibrant, with a creamy pesto that perfectly balances the juicy burst of cherry tomatoes.

Ingredients

1 large zucchini, spiralized

1/2 cup cherry tomatoes, halved

2 tbsp basil pesto (preferably homemade)

1 tbsp olive oil

Salt and pepper to taste

Instructions

Heat olive oil in a skillet over medium heat.

Add spiralized zucchini and sauté lightly for 1-2 minutes.

Toss with pesto and cherry tomatoes, seasoning with salt and pepper.

Health Benefits: Zucchini noodles are low in carbs and high in fiber, while basil and olive oil provide antioxidants and healthy fats.

Chickpea and Avocado Salad with Cucumber and Mint

Crisp, cooling, and refreshing, with creamy avocado and a hint of mint to lift the flavors.

Ingredients

1 cup chickpeas, cooked

1/2 avocado, diced

1/2 cucumber, diced

1 tbsp fresh mint, chopped

Juice of 1/2 lemon

Salt and pepper to taste

Instructions

In a large bowl, combine chickpeas, avocado, cucumber, and mint.

Drizzle with lemon juice, and season with salt and pepper, tossing to combine.

Health Benefits: Chickpeas offer protein and fiber for energy, while avocado provides heart-healthy fats essential for cellular function.

Cauliflower Fried Rice with Edamame and Carrots

A light, savory "rice" dish with a hint of ginger, colorful veggies, and a satisfyingly crisp texture.

Ingredients

2 cups cauliflower rice

1/2 cup shelled edamame

1/4 cup diced carrots

1 green onion, chopped

1 tbsp coconut aminos or low-sodium soy sauce

1 tsp grated ginger

1 tsp sesame oil

Instructions

Heat sesame oil in a skillet and add cauliflower rice, carrots, and edamame.

Sauté for 5-6 minutes until veggies are tender. Stir in green onions, ginger, and coconut aminos.

Health Benefits: Cauliflower is rich in fiber and antioxidants, and edamame provides protein and essential amino acids.

Spinach and Lentil Stew with Garlic and Tomatoes

Warm, earthy, and comforting, with the richness of lentils and the tang of tomatoes.

Ingredients

1 cup cooked lentils

1 cup fresh spinach

1/2 cup diced tomatoes

2 cloves garlic, minced

1 tbsp olive oil

Salt and pepper to taste

Instructions

Heat olive oil in a pot and sauté garlic until fragrant.

Add tomatoes, spinach, and lentils, cooking for 5 minutes until spinach wilts.

Season with salt and pepper, and serve warm.

Health Benefits: Lentils are a powerhouse of iron and fiber, supporting energy levels and blood sugar stability.

Avocado and Veggie Spring Rolls with Almond Dipping Sauce

Crisp, colorful, and light, with creamy avocado and a hint of nutty sweetness from the dipping sauce.

Ingredients

Rice paper wrappers

1/2 avocado, sliced

1/4 cup shredded carrots

1/4 cup sliced bell pepper

Fresh basil and cilantro leaves

Almond Sauce: 1 tbsp almond butter, 1 tbsp soy sauce, 1 tsp honey, water to thin

Instructions

Dip rice paper wrappers in warm water to soften. Lay on a flat surface.

Place avocado, carrots, bell pepper, basil, and cilantro in the center.

Roll tightly, folding in the sides.

For the almond sauce, mix almond butter, soy sauce, honey, and water until smooth.

Health Benefits: Fresh veggies provide essential vitamins, while almond butter adds healthy fats and protein for satiety.

These recipes are crafted to boost your mitochondrial health while keeping your energy levels balanced throughout the day. Let me know if you'd like to explore more meal ideas!

Snacks Recipes For Mitochondrial Health

Here's an enhanced version of Mitochondria-Supporting Afternoon Snacks with improved step-by-step instructions for clarity and ease of preparation. Each snack now includes sensory details along with instructions for each step.

Cucumber and Hummus Bites

Crisp, cool cucumber pairs with smooth, garlicky hummus for a refreshing, savory bite.

Ingredients

1 cucumber, sliced into 1/4-inch rounds

1/2 cup hummus

1/4 tsp paprika or fresh chopped parsley for garnish

Instructions

Wash and dry the cucumber, then slice it into rounds about 1/4 inch thick.

Place a small dollop (about 1 tsp) of hummus on each cucumber slice.

Sprinkle each bite with a pinch of paprika or garnish with parsley.

Health Benefits: Cucumber hydrates, and hummus adds fiber and protein, helping sustain energy.

Apple Slices with Almond Butter

Crisp, juicy apple slices topped with rich, creamy almond butter, with a hint of cinnamon warmth.

Ingredients

1 apple, sliced into wedges

2 tbsp almond butter

1/4 tsp cinnamon (optional)

Instructions

Core and slice the apple into thin wedges.

Spread a thin layer of almond butter over each apple slice.

Sprinkle with cinnamon if desired.

Health Benefits: Apples provide fiber, while almond butter offers healthy fats, helping stabilize blood sugar.

Energy Balls with Oats and Coconut

Soft, chewy, nutty bites with a hint of coconut sweetness.

Ingredients

1/2 cup rolled oats

1/4 cup almond butter

1/4 cup shredded coconut

1 tbsp honey or maple syrup

Instructions

In a medium bowl, mix the oats, almond butter, shredded coconut, and honey or maple syrup until fully combined.

Roll the mixture into small balls (about 1 inch in diameter).

Place the energy balls on a plate, cover, and refrigerate for at least 30 minutes.

Health Benefits: Oats provide fiber, while coconut adds MCTs for quick energy. Almond butter adds protein and healthy fats.

Greek Yogurt with Berries and Flaxseed

Creamy yogurt with bursts of sweet berries and nutty flaxseed crunch.

Ingredients

1/2 cup plain Greek yogurt

1/4 cup fresh mixed berries

1 tsp ground flaxseed

Instructions

Spoon the Greek yogurt into a small bowl.

Scatter the mixed berries over the yogurt.

Sprinkle with flaxseed for added texture and flavor.

Health Benefits: Yogurt offers protein and probiotics, while berries and flaxseed provide antioxidants and omega-3s.

Homemade Kale Chips

Crispy, light, and slightly salty with an earthy, fresh aroma.

Ingredients

1 cup kale leaves, stemmed and torn

1 tbsp olive oil

Sea salt, to taste

Instructions

Preheat your oven to 300°F (150°C).

Rinse the kale, dry well, and place in a large bowl. Drizzle with olive oil and toss to coat.

Arrange the kale in a single layer on a baking sheet, sprinkle with sea salt, and bake for 10-15 minutes, or until crisp.

Health Benefits: Kale is packed with antioxidants, supporting cellular health.

Carrot Sticks with Fresh Guacamole

Sweet, crisp carrots with smooth, creamy, and tangy guacamole.

Ingredients

2 large carrots, peeled and cut into sticks

1/2 avocado

1/2 lime, juiced

Salt, to taste

Instructions

Cut the avocado, remove the pit, and scoop the flesh into a bowl. Mash with a fork until smooth.

Add lime juice and salt to taste, mixing well.

Serve with the carrot sticks.

Health Benefits: Carrots add beta-carotene, while avocado provides healthy fats and antioxidants.

Spiced Roasted Chickpeas

Crispy, warm, and slightly smoky with a savory aroma.

Ingredients

1 cup cooked chickpeas

1 tbsp olive oil

1/2 tsp paprika, 1/2 tsp garlic powder, pinch of salt

Instructions

Preheat oven to 400°F (200°C).

Rinse and drain the chickpeas, then pat them dry.

Toss the chickpeas with olive oil and spices. Spread on a baking sheet and bake for 20-25 minutes, stirring halfway.

Health Benefits: Chickpeas are high in fiber and protein, which aids satiety and energy levels.

Avocado and Tomato on Toast

Creamy avocado with juicy tomato on a crunchy, nutty slice of whole-grain toast.

Ingredients

1 slice whole-grain bread, toasted

1/2 avocado, mashed

2-3 cherry tomatoes, sliced

Salt and pepper to taste

Instructions

Spread mashed avocado over the toasted bread.

Arrange cherry tomato slices on top and season with salt and pepper.

Health Benefits: Whole grains support heart health, while avocado offers healthy fats beneficial for cell health.

9. Blueberry Chia Pudding

Creamy, cool pudding with bursts of blueberry sweetness and slight chia crunch.

Ingredients

1/4 cup chia seeds

1 cup almond milk

1/4 cup blueberries

1 tsp honey or maple syrup

Instructions

Mix chia seeds, almond milk, and honey in a jar or bowl.

Stir well, cover, and refrigerate overnight.

Before serving, add fresh blueberries.

Health Benefits: Chia seeds are high in omega-3s, which are crucial for mitochondrial function.

10. Sweet Potato Fries with Smoked Paprika

Crispy on the outside, tender inside, with a subtly sweet and smoky flavor.

Ingredients

1 medium sweet potato, cut into fries

1 tbsp olive oil

1/2 tsp smoked paprika

Salt, to taste

Instructions

Preheat the oven to 400°F (200°C).

Toss sweet potato fries in olive oil, paprika, and salt.

Spread in a single layer on a baking sheet and bake for 20-25 minutes, flipping halfway.

Health Benefits: Sweet potatoes provide beta-carotene and fiber, fueling sustained energy for cells.

These nutrient-rich, mitochondria-supporting snacks are designed to boost your energy and health in a tasty, accessible way! Let me know if you need further adjustments or additional recipes.

Lunch Recipes For Mitochondrial Health

Here's a selection of Restorative Dinner Recipes designed for mitochondrial support. These recipes focus on nutrient-dense ingredients that promote energy production and cellular health, describing the sensory experience and giving thorough step-by-step preparation instructions.

Garlic & Herb Salmon with Roasted Vegetables

Succulent, flaky salmon with a fresh herb aroma, paired with tender, caramelized vegetables.

Ingredients

2 salmon fillets

1 tbsp olive oil

2 cloves garlic, minced

1 tsp fresh rosemary and thyme, chopped

Salt and pepper, to taste

1 cup broccoli florets

1/2 cup sliced bell peppers

1/2 cup sliced zucchini

Instructions

Preheat oven to 400°F (200°C).

In a small bowl, mix olive oil, garlic, rosemary, thyme, salt, and pepper.

Place salmon and vegetables on a baking sheet, brushing the salmon with the oil mixture.

Roast for 15-20 minutes until the salmon flakes easily.

Health Benefits: Omega-3s in salmon reduce inflammation, supporting mitochondrial efficiency.

Lemon Rosemary Chicken with Sweet Potato Mash

Juicy chicken with bright citrus and herb notes, paired with creamy, naturally sweet mash.

Ingredients

2 chicken breasts

1 lemon, zested and juiced

1 tsp rosemary

1 tbsp olive oil

2 medium sweet potatoes, peeled and cubed

Salt and pepper, to taste

Instructions

Marinate chicken in lemon juice, zest, rosemary, olive oil, salt, and pepper for 30 minutes.

Bake at 375°F for 25 minutes.

Boil sweet potatoes until tender, mash, and season with a pinch of salt.

Health Benefits: Sweet potatoes offer beta-carotene and fiber, fueling sustained energy release.

Quinoa Stuffed Bell Peppers

Soft, sweet bell peppers filled with savory quinoa and fresh herbs.

Ingredients

4 bell peppers, tops cut off and seeds removed

1 cup cooked quinoa

1/4 cup diced tomatoes

1/4 cup black beans

Fresh basil, chopped

Salt and pepper, to taste

Instructions

Preheat oven to 375°F.

Mix quinoa, tomatoes, beans, basil, salt, and pepper. Fill each pepper with the mixture.

Bake for 25-30 minutes until peppers are tender.

Health Benefits: Quinoa provides protein and fiber, promoting stable blood sugar.

Zucchini Noodles with Pesto and Cherry Tomatoes

Light, crisp zucchini noodles with the vibrant aroma of basil pesto and juicy tomatoes.

Ingredients

2 medium zucchinis, spiralized

1 cup cherry tomatoes, halved

1/4 cup fresh basil pesto

Instructions

Lightly sauté zucchini noodles in a skillet until warm but firm.

Stir in pesto and cherry tomatoes, and cook for another 1-2 minutes.

Health Benefits: Zucchini is low in carbs and high in antioxidants, aiding cellular protection.

Cauliflower and Chickpea Curry

A creamy, aromatic dish with warming spices and tender vegetables.

Ingredients

1 cup cauliflower florets

1/2 cup chickpeas, cooked

1/2 onion, diced

1 garlic clove, minced

1 tsp curry powder

1/2 cup coconut milk

Instructions

Sauté onion and garlic until translucent, then add curry powder.

Add cauliflower, chickpeas, and coconut milk; simmer until cauliflower is tender.

Health Benefits: Coconut milk provides healthy fats, while chickpeas add protein and fiber for satiety.

Spinach and Mushroom Stuffed Chicken Breast

Juicy chicken with earthy mushrooms and vibrant spinach filling.

Ingredients

2 chicken breasts, butterflied

1 cup spinach, chopped

1/2 cup mushrooms, diced

1 garlic clove, minced

Instructions

Sauté garlic, mushrooms, and spinach until softened.

Stuff chicken with the mixture, secure with toothpicks, and bake at 375°F for 25 minutes.

Health Benefits: Spinach and mushrooms offer antioxidants and B vitamins, crucial for cellular health.

Baked Cod with Lemon and Asparagus

Delicate, flaky cod with fresh citrus and tender asparagus.

Ingredients

2 cod fillets

1 lemon, sliced

1 cup asparagus spears

Salt and pepper, to taste

Instructions

Place cod and asparagus on a baking sheet, topping with lemon slices.

Season with salt and pepper and bake at 400°F for 15 minutes.

Health Benefits: Cod is high in protein and low in fat, with omega-3s for cell function.

Stuffed Portobello Mushrooms with Spinach and Feta

Juicy mushrooms with a creamy, tangy filling of spinach and feta.

Ingredients

4 large portobello mushrooms

1 cup spinach, chopped

1/4 cup feta cheese, crumbled

Instructions

Preheat oven to 375°F.

Remove mushroom stems, fill with spinach and feta, and bake for 20 minutes.

Health Benefits: Mushrooms provide B vitamins, while spinach and feta offer iron and calcium.

Turkey and Vegetable Stir-Fry

Tender turkey with vibrant, crisp veggies and a hint of ginger and garlic.

Ingredients

1/2 lb ground turkey

1 cup mixed bell peppers, sliced

1/2 cup snap peas

1 garlic clove, minced

1 tsp ginger, grated

Instructions

Sauté garlic and ginger, then add ground turkey until cooked through.

Add bell peppers and snap peas, cook until tender-crisp.

Health Benefits: Turkey is rich in protein, while bell peppers add vitamin C, supporting immune function.

Lentil and Vegetable Stew

Hearty, warm, and comforting with rich flavors of earthy lentils and fresh vegetables.

Ingredients

1/2 cup lentils, rinsed

1 carrot, diced

1 celery stalk, diced

1/2 onion, diced

1 cup vegetable broth

Instructions

Sauté onion, carrot, and celery until softened.

Add lentils and broth, bring to a boil, then simmer until lentils are tender.

Health Benefits: Lentils offer plant-based protein and iron, aiding energy production.

These restorative dinners provide nourishing support for mitochondrial health, with each dish crafted to fuel your cells and optimize energy production naturally. Let me know if you'd like additional recipes or specific details on any dish!

Lunch Recipes For Mitochondrial Health

Here are Decadent Dessert Recipes for the Mitochondria Diet, which feature ingredients that support mitochondrial health and are designed to satisfy your sweet cravings without compromising on nutrition. These desserts are nutrient-dense, rich in antioxidants, healthy fats, and essential vitamins, which contribute to energy production and cellular health.

Dark Chocolate Avocado Mousse

A smooth, creamy mousse with rich cocoa flavor and a hint of sweetness.

Ingredients

1 ripe avocado, peeled and pitted

1/4 cup unsweetened cocoa powder

2 tbsp honey or maple syrup

1 tsp vanilla extract

1/4 cup almond milk

Instructions

Blend all ingredients in a food processor until smooth and creamy.

Chill for at least 30 minutes before serving.

Health Benefits: Avocado is rich in monounsaturated fats, supporting cell membranes and mitochondrial function, while cocoa provides antioxidants.

Chia Seed Pudding with Berries

A refreshing, slightly sweet pudding with the crunch of chia seeds and juicy berries.

Ingredients

1/4 cup chia seeds

1 cup unsweetened almond milk

1 tbsp honey or agave

1/2 tsp vanilla extract

Fresh mixed berries

Instructions

Combine chia seeds, almond milk, honey, and vanilla in a bowl.

Stir well, cover, and refrigerate for at least 4 hours or overnight.

Top with fresh berries before serving.

Health Benefits: Chia seeds are rich in omega-3 fatty acids, supporting mitochondrial health, and berries provide antioxidants for cell protection.

Coconut Almond Energy Balls

Bite-sized, chewy, and nutty with a hint of sweetness from coconut and almond.

Ingredients

1/2 cup almond butter

1/2 cup shredded coconut

1/4 cup raw almonds, chopped

2 tbsp honey or maple syrup

1/4 tsp vanilla extract

Instructions

Combine all ingredients in a bowl and mix well.

Roll mixture into small balls and refrigerate for 1 hour.

Health Benefits: Almonds provide healthy fats and vitamin E, which support mitochondrial function, while coconut offers medium-chain triglycerides (MCTs) for quick energy.

Baked Apple Cinnamon Crisps

Warm, cinnamon-spiced apples with a crisp texture, perfect for a sweet yet light dessert.

Ingredients

2 apples, thinly sliced

1 tsp ground cinnamon

1 tbsp coconut oil

Instructions

Preheat oven to 350°F (175°C).

Toss apple slices with cinnamon and coconut oil.

Arrange on a baking sheet and bake for 25-30 minutes until crisp.

Health Benefits: Apples provide fiber and antioxidants, while coconut oil offers healthy fats that support cell function.

Pumpkin Spice Coconut Bars

Soft, spiced bars with a rich pumpkin flavor and a coconutty finish.

Ingredients

1/2 cup canned pumpkin

1/4 cup coconut flour

2 eggs

1/4 cup honey

1 tsp pumpkin spice

Instructions

Preheat oven to 350°F (175°C).

Mix all ingredients together in a bowl.

Pour mixture into a baking pan and bake for 20-25 minutes.

Health Benefits: Pumpkin is high in beta-carotene, supporting mitochondrial health and offering antioxidants.

Blueberry Lemon Sorbet

A refreshing, tart-sweet sorbet with the vibrant flavor of fresh blueberries and zesty lemon.

Ingredients

2 cups fresh or frozen blueberries

1/4 cup lemon juice

1 tbsp honey or agave

1/4 cup water

Instructions

Blend all ingredients in a food processor until smooth.

Freeze the mixture for 4-6 hours, stirring every hour.

Health Benefits: Blueberries are packed with antioxidants, while lemon provides vitamin C to support mitochondrial function and energy production.

Cacao and Nut Butter Brownies

Fudgy, rich brownies with deep cocoa flavor and creamy nut butter swirls.

Ingredients

1/2 cup almond butter

1/4 cup unsweetened cocoa powder

2 eggs

1/4 cup honey or maple syrup

1/2 tsp vanilla extract

Instructions

Preheat oven to 350°F (175°C).

Mix all ingredients in a bowl until smooth.

Pour into a baking dish and bake for 20-25 minutes.

Health Benefits: Almond butter provides healthy fats and protein, supporting mitochondrial function, while cacao is rich in flavonoids for cellular health.

Avocado Lime Popsicles

Creamy avocado with a refreshing lime tang makes a perfect sweet treat on a hot day.

Ingredients

1 ripe avocado

1/2 cup coconut milk

2 tbsp honey or maple syrup

1 tbsp lime juice

Instructions

Blend all ingredients in a food processor until smooth.

Pour into popsicle molds and freeze for 4-6 hours.

Health Benefits: Avocados provide monounsaturated fats that support cellular health, while lime juice offers vitamin C, boosting energy production.

Almond Flour Chocolate Chip Cookies

Chewy cookies with rich chocolate chips and the nutty flavor of almond flour.

Ingredients

1 cup almond flour

1/4 cup coconut oil, melted

1/4 cup honey

1/2 cup dark chocolate chips

Instructions

Preheat oven to 350°F (175°C).

Mix almond flour, coconut oil, and honey.

Fold in chocolate chips and drop spoonfuls of dough on a baking sheet.

Bake for 10-12 minutes.

Health Benefits: Almond flour provides magnesium and vitamin E, which are crucial for mitochondrial health, while dark chocolate offers antioxidants.

Mango Coconut Parfait

A layered dessert with creamy coconut yogurt and sweet, tropical mango.

Ingredients

1 cup coconut yogurt

1 ripe mango, diced

1/4 cup shredded coconut

Instructions

Layer coconut yogurt, diced mango, and shredded coconut in glasses.

Chill in the fridge for 1 hour before serving.

Health Benefits: Coconut provides medium-chain triglycerides (MCTs) for fast energy, and mango is high in vitamin A for cellular repair.

These desserts support mitochondrial health with antioxidants, healthy fats, and essential vitamins that help power your cells. They are delicious, nourishing treats to indulge in while supporting overall wellness.

Meat and Poultry Recipes For Mitochondrial Health

Here are meat and poultry recipes for a Mitochondria Diet, designed to nourish and support mitochondrial health. These dishes are crafted to deliver essential nutrients, including healthy fats, proteins, vitamins, and minerals that can aid in optimal mitochondrial function, boost energy production, and support overall cellular health.

Grilled Chicken with Avocado and Spinach Salad

A fresh, vibrant dish with tender grilled chicken paired with creamy avocado and earthy spinach.

Ingredients

2 chicken breasts

1 avocado, sliced

4 cups spinach

1/4 cup olive oil

1 tbsp lemon juice

Salt and pepper to taste

Instructions

Preheat the grill to medium-high heat.

Season chicken breasts with salt, pepper, and a drizzle of olive oil.

Grill chicken for 6-8 minutes per side until fully cooked.

Toss spinach, avocado, olive oil, and lemon juice in a bowl.

Slice chicken and serve over salad.

Health Benefits: Avocados provide healthy fats that support mitochondrial membranes, and spinach is rich in antioxidants, promoting cellular repair.

Turmeric Chicken Stir-Fry

A fragrant, spiced stir-fry with tender chicken and the warm, earthy flavor of turmeric.

Ingredients

2 chicken breasts, cut into strips

1 tbsp turmeric

1 tbsp olive oil

1 bell pepper, sliced

1/2 onion, sliced

1/4 cup coconut milk

Salt and pepper to taste

Instructions

Heat olive oil in a pan over medium heat.

Add chicken strips, salt, pepper, and turmeric, cooking until golden brown.

Add bell pepper and onion, stir-frying for 3-5 minutes.

Pour in coconut milk and simmer for 3 minutes.

Health Benefits: Turmeric is a powerful anti-inflammatory that supports mitochondrial function, while coconut milk offers medium-chain triglycerides for fast energy.

Salmon with Lemon and Dill

A light, zesty salmon fillet with a delicate, flaky texture, accented by fresh lemon and dill.

Ingredients

2 salmon fillets

1 lemon, sliced

2 tbsp fresh dill

1 tbsp olive oil

Salt and pepper to taste

Instructions

Preheat oven to 375°F (190°C).

Place salmon on a baking sheet, drizzle with olive oil, and season with salt and pepper.

Top with lemon slices and fresh dill.

Bake for 12-15 minutes, until salmon is cooked through.

Health Benefits: Salmon is rich in omega-3 fatty acids, supporting mitochondrial health and reducing inflammation.

Grass-fed beef Stir-Fry with Broccoli

Tender grass-fed beef stir-fried with crunchy, nutrient-packed broccoli for a satisfying, savory meal.

Ingredients

1 lb grass-fed beef, thinly sliced

1 cup broccoli florets

1 tbsp sesame oil

1 tbsp soy sauce (low sodium)

2 garlic cloves, minced

Instructions

Heat sesame oil in a pan over medium-high heat.

Add beef and cook until browned.

Stir in garlic and broccoli, sautéing until tender.

Add soy sauce and cook for an additional 2-3 minutes.

Health Benefits: Grass-fed beef is high in conjugated linoleic acid (CLA), which helps reduce inflammation and support mitochondrial health.

Chicken and Zucchini Noodles

A low-carb, fresh dish with tender chicken paired with zucchini noodles, offering a light but filling meal.

Ingredients

2 chicken breasts, grilled and sliced

2 zucchinis, spiralized into noodles

1 tbsp olive oil

1/4 cup grated parmesan

1 tbsp fresh basil

Instructions

Sauté zucchini noodles in olive oil for 2-3 minutes until tender.

Add sliced chicken and toss together.

Top with parmesan and fresh basil.

Health Benefits: Zucchini is rich in antioxidants, and chicken provides lean protein that supports muscle and mitochondrial function.

Lamb Chops with Mint Pesto

Juicy lamb chops are served with a refreshing, fragrant mint pesto that complements the rich meat.

Ingredients

4 lamb chops

1/2 cup fresh mint leaves

1/4 cup olive oil

1 tbsp lemon juice

Salt and pepper to taste

Instructions

Season lamb chops with salt and pepper, then grill or sear them to your desired doneness.

For pesto, blend mint, olive oil, lemon juice, and salt in a food processor.

Serve lamb with a drizzle of mint pesto on top.

Health Benefits: Lamb provides zinc and iron, crucial for mitochondrial energy production, while mint offers antioxidants and digestive support.

Chicken and Sweet Potato Skillet

A one-pan meal with juicy chicken and soft, roasted sweet potatoes that balance savory and sweet flavors.

Ingredients

2 chicken breasts, cut into cubes

2 sweet potatoes, diced

1 tbsp olive oil

1 tsp paprika

1/2 tsp cumin

Salt and pepper to taste

Instructions

Heat olive oil in a skillet over medium heat.

Add chicken cubes, season with paprika, cumin, salt, and pepper, and cook until browned.

Add diced sweet potatoes, cover, and cook for 10-12 minutes until tender.

Health Benefits: Sweet potatoes are rich in vitamin A, promoting mitochondrial health, while chicken provides essential protein for cellular repair.

Turkey Meatballs with Cauliflower Rice

Lean turkey meatballs served with light, fluffy cauliflower rice for a delicious, low-carb meal.

Ingredients

1 lb ground turkey

1/4 cup almond flour

1 egg

1 head of cauliflower, riced

1 tbsp olive oil

1 tsp dried oregano

Salt and pepper to taste

Instructions

Mix ground turkey, almond flour, egg, oregano, salt, and pepper.

Form into meatballs and bake at 375°F (190°C) for 20 minutes.

Sauté cauliflower rice in olive oil until tender and serve with meatballs.

Health Benefits: Turkey is an excellent source of lean protein, while cauliflower rice provides a low-carb, high-antioxidant alternative to grains.

Grilled Chicken with Asparagus and Lemon

Light, zesty grilled chicken paired with crispy asparagus and a bright lemony finish.

Ingredients

2 chicken breasts

1 bunch asparagus, trimmed

1 lemon, sliced

1 tbsp olive oil

Salt and pepper to taste

Instructions

Preheat the grill to medium-high heat.

Season chicken breasts and asparagus with olive oil, salt, and pepper.

Grill chicken for 6-8 minutes per side, and grill asparagus for 3-4 minutes.

Serve chicken with asparagus and lemon slices.

Health Benefits: Asparagus is high in folate, supporting cellular energy, and chicken provides protein for muscle and mitochondrial repair.

Beef and Veggie Stir-Fry

A savory stir-fry with tender strips of beef and crunchy vegetables, lightly seasoned for a balanced meal.

Ingredients

1 lb grass-fed beef, sliced thinly

1 bell pepper, sliced

1 cup snap peas

1 tbsp olive oil

2 tbsp soy sauce (low sodium)

1 garlic clove, minced

Instructions

Heat olive oil in a pan over medium-high heat.

Add beef and cook until browned, then add garlic and vegetables.

Stir-fry for 5-7 minutes, then add soy sauce and cook for 2 more minutes.

Health Benefits: Grass-fed beef is rich in CLA, supporting mitochondrial function, and vegetables provide essential antioxidants for cellular health.

These meat and poultry recipes provide a healthy mix of proteins, healthy fats, and vitamins that fuel your body and support mitochondrial health. By focusing on lean meats, healthy oils, and nutrient-dense vegetables,

Note: Red meat are said to be avoided, but for meat lovers who enjoy meat in every meal can actually incorporate these satisfactory meat recipes.

Smoothie and Salad Recipes For Mitochondrial Health

Here are mitochondria-boosting smoothie and salad recipes, each crafted to deliver vibrant flavors and textures while supporting cellular health. Every recipe is designed with nutrient-rich ingredients that can optimize mitochondrial function, providing antioxidants, healthy fats, and essential vitamins.

Green Power Smoothie

This smoothie is creamy and vibrant, with a slightly sweet, earthy flavor and a fresh, green aroma.

Ingredients

1 cup spinach

1/2 avocado

1/2 cup pineapple

1/2 cup coconut water

1 tbsp chia seeds

Ice cubes

Instruction

Add all ingredients to a blender.

Blend on high until smooth and creamy.

Pour into a glass and enjoy immediately.

Health Benefit: Rich in antioxidants and healthy fats, this smoothie supports mitochondrial function and energy production.

Berry Beet Smoothie

A deep purple smoothie with a tangy, sweet taste and a rich, earthy aroma from the beets.

Ingredients

1/2 cup blueberries

1/2 cup strawberries

1 small cooked beet

1/2 cup almond milk

1 tbsp hemp seeds

Instruction

Combine all ingredients in a blender.

Blend until smooth.

Serve chilled, garnished with a few extra berries if desired.

Health Benefit: Packed with anthocyanins and nitrates, which can improve blood flow and mitochondrial efficiency.

Citrus Sunshine Smoothie

Bright and zesty, with a refreshing citrus aroma and smooth, creamy texture.

Ingredients

1 orange, peeled

1/2 lemon, juiced

1 banana

1/2 cup plain Greek yogurt

1 tbsp flaxseed

Instruction

Place all ingredients in a blender.

Blend until well combined and smooth.

Serve immediately for optimal freshness.

Health Benefit: The citrus and yogurt provide vitamin C and probiotics, both essential for mitochondrial and immune support.

Turmeric Mango Smoothie

A sweet, tropical flavor with a golden hue, and a hint of warmth from turmeric.

Ingredients

1/2 cup mango chunks

1/2 banana

1 cup coconut milk

1/2 tsp turmeric

1/4 tsp black pepper

Instruction

Blend all ingredients until smooth.

Adjust thickness with more coconut milk, if desired.

Serve and enjoy.

Health Benefit: Turmeric contains curcumin, a powerful anti-inflammatory that supports mitochondrial resilience.

Kale and Pomegranate Salad

Crisp and vibrant, with a pop of sweetness from the pomegranate seeds and a tangy dressing.

Ingredients

2 cups chopped kale

1/4 cup pomegranate seeds

1/4 cup walnuts, chopped

2 tbsp olive oil

1 tbsp apple cider vinegar

Instruction

Massage the kale with olive oil until softened.

Add pomegranate seeds and walnuts.

Drizzle with apple cider vinegar, toss, and serve.

Health Benefit: Rich in antioxidants and healthy fats, this salad helps reduce oxidative stress on mitochondria.

Spinach and Blueberry Salad

Fresh and sweet with a soft crunch, showcasing a balance of spinach's earthiness and blueberry's sweetness.

Ingredients

2 cups baby spinach

1/2 cup blueberries

1 tbsp sunflower seeds

2 tbsp balsamic vinaigrette

Instruction

Combine spinach, blueberries, and sunflower seeds.

Drizzle with balsamic vinaigrette and toss gently.

Health Benefit: High in antioxidants and vitamins, this salad supports mitochondrial health and combats oxidative damage.

Cucumber Avocado Smoothie

Cool, refreshing, and creamy with a subtle hint of cucumber freshness.

Ingredients

1/2 cucumber, peeled and sliced

1/2 avocado

1/2 cup coconut water

Juice of 1 lime

Ice cubes

Instruction

Blend all ingredients until smooth.

Serve cold.

Health Benefit: This hydrating smoothie provides potassium and electrolytes that aid cellular function.

Orange Ginger Salad

Zesty, with a bit of a spicy kick from ginger and a refreshing crunch.

Ingredients

1 large orange, segmented

1/2 tsp grated ginger

1/2 cup arugula

1 tbsp pumpkin seeds

Instruction

Arrange arugula, orange segments, and pumpkin seeds.

Sprinkle with ginger and serve.

Health Benefit: Rich in vitamin C and anti-inflammatory compounds, aiding in energy production and immune health.

Pineapple Mint Smoothie

A sweet tropical flavor, brightened by mint, creating a refreshing and energizing drink.

Ingredients

1/2 cup pineapple chunks

1/4 cup fresh mint leaves

1 cup unsweetened almond milk

Ice cubes

Instruction

Blend all ingredients until smooth.

Pour and enjoy immediately.

Health Benefit: Pineapple offers digestive enzymes, and mint helps soothe digestion, supporting nutrient absorption.

Red Pepper and Avocado Salad

Description: Crunchy, creamy, with a slightly sweet and smoky flavor from roasted red peppers.

Ingredients

1/2 red bell pepper, sliced

1/2 avocado, diced

1 cup mixed greens

2 tbsp olive oil

1 tbsp lemon juice

Instruction

Toss greens, red pepper, and avocado.

Drizzle with olive oil and lemon juice.

Health Benefit: Packed with vitamins A and C, this salad boosts antioxidant defenses and supports skin health.

Each of these recipes is designed not only to satisfy taste buds but also to provide essential nutrients that fuel and protect mitochondria, supporting sustained energy and cellular health.

Chapter Four

14-day meal plan

Here's a 14-day meal plan for a mitochondria-supportive diet. This plan emphasizes foods high in antioxidants, essential vitamins, minerals, and healthy fats that enhance mitochondrial function and energy production.

Day 1

Breakfast: Green Power Smoothie (spinach, avocado, pineapple, coconut water, chia seeds)

Lunch: Spinach and Blueberry Salad (spinach, blueberries, sunflower seeds, balsamic vinaigrette)

Dinner: Salmon with Roasted Vegetables (broccoli, bell peppers, and carrots with olive oil)

Snack: Almonds and a piece of dark chocolate

Day 2

Breakfast: Citrus Sunshine Smoothie (orange, lemon, banana, Greek yogurt, flaxseed)

Lunch: Quinoa and Roasted Beet Salad (quinoa, roasted beets, arugula, pumpkin seeds)

Dinner: Chicken with Garlic and Asparagus (grilled chicken breast, asparagus, garlic, olive oil)

Snack: Greek yogurt with fresh berries

Day 3

Breakfast: Turmeric Mango Smoothie (mango, banana, coconut milk, turmeric, black pepper)

Lunch: Kale and Pomegranate Salad (kale, pomegranate seeds, walnuts, apple cider vinegar)

Dinner: Grilled Tuna with Steamed Green Beans and Sweet Potatoes

Snack: Celery sticks with almond butter

Day 4

Breakfast: Overnight Oats with Chia Seeds, Blueberries, and Almond Milk

Lunch: Lentil and Vegetable Soup (lentils, carrots, celery, onions)

Dinner: Baked Cod with Lemon and Roasted Brussels Sprouts

Snack: Handful of walnuts

Day 5

Breakfast: Pineapple Mint Smoothie (pineapple, mint, almond milk)

Lunch: Zucchini Noodles with Avocado Pesto (zucchini noodles, avocado, basil, olive oil)

Dinner: Turkey Meatballs with Cauliflower Mash

Snack: Sliced apple with a sprinkle of cinnamon

Day 6

Breakfast: Greek Yogurt with Honey, Walnuts, and Fresh Raspberries

Lunch: Chickpea and Cucumber Salad (chickpeas, cucumber, tomatoes, parsley, olive oil)

Dinner: Grilled Shrimp Skewers with Mixed Veggies (bell peppers, onions, cherry tomatoes)

Snack: Handful of mixed berries

Day 7

Breakfast: Cucumber Avocado Smoothie (cucumber, avocado, coconut water, lime)

Lunch: Roasted Veggie Wrap (whole grain wrap, roasted vegetables, hummus)

Dinner: Baked Lemon Chicken with Sautéed Spinach

Snack: Carrot sticks with guacamole

Day 8

Breakfast: Chia Seed Pudding with Almond Milk and Strawberries

Lunch: Sweet Potato and Black Bean Salad (sweet potato, black beans, spinach, lime dressing)

Dinner: Grilled Salmon with Asparagus and Brown Rice

Snack: Sliced bell peppers with hummus

Day 9

Breakfast: Berry Beet Smoothie (blueberries, strawberries, beet, almond milk, hemp seeds)

Lunch: Quinoa Salad with Mixed Greens, Feta, and Pumpkin Seeds

Dinner: Beef Stir-Fry with Broccoli, Carrots, and Cauliflower Rice

Snack: Coconut yogurt with chia seeds

Day 10

Breakfast: Scrambled Eggs with Spinach and Tomatoes

Lunch: Mediterranean Chickpea Bowl (chickpeas, cucumber, tomatoes, olives, feta)

Dinner: Miso Soup with Tofu and Seaweed, Side of Steamed Edamame

Snack: Cucumber slices with sea salt

Day 11

Breakfast: Green Smoothie Bowl (spinach, banana, almond milk, topped with granola)

Lunch: Grilled Chicken Salad with Mixed Greens and Avocado

Dinner: Seared Tuna with Cabbage and Carrot Slaw

Snack: Handful of pistachios

Day 12

Breakfast: Mango Chia Pudding (mango, chia seeds, almond milk)

Lunch: Cauliflower Tabouleh (cauliflower, parsley, tomatoes, lemon)

Dinner: Spaghetti Squash with Marinara and Turkey Meatballs

Snack: Celery with almond butter

Day 13

Breakfast: Apple Cinnamon Overnight Oats (oats, apple, cinnamon, almond milk)

Lunch: Spinach, Kale, and Pomegranate Salad with a Citrus Vinaigrette

Dinner: Shrimp Stir-Fry with Zucchini Noodles

Snack: Mixed berries with a sprinkle of hemp seeds

Breakfast: Orange Ginger Smoothie (orange, ginger, banana, almond milk)

Lunch: Roasted Veggie Power Bowl (sweet potato, quinoa, broccoli, tahini dressing)

Dinner: Baked Cod with a Side of Sautéed Greens

Snack: Small piece of dark chocolate and walnuts

This meal plan is packed with nutrient-dense ingredients to support mitochondrial function, improve energy, and help manage oxidative stress. By incorporating antioxidant-rich foods, lean proteins, and healthy fats, these meals contribute to overall cellular health and vitality.

Daily Routines to Support Mitochondrial Health

Supporting mitochondrial health with daily routines can significantly enhance your energy, overall vitality, and cellular resilience. Here's a comprehensive guide to routines that promote optimal mitochondrial function:

1. Nourishing Morning Habits

- ***Hydrate First Thing:*** Start the day with a glass of water to rehydrate cells and support detoxification. Adding a splash of lemon provides vitamin C, which helps protect mitochondria from oxidative stress.

- ***Light Movement or Stretching:*** Gentle morning exercise activates circulation and can stimulate mitochondria in muscles. Activities like yoga or a short walk boost blood flow, oxygen delivery, and mitochondrial health.

- **Breakfast Rich in Healthy Fats and Low Glycemic Foods:** Foods like avocado, nuts, seeds, and berries are high in antioxidants, healthy fats, and nutrients that support mitochondrial energy production and reduce inflammation.

2. Mindful Midday Routine

- ***Take Breaks for Movement:*** Sitting for prolonged periods can reduce mitochondrial efficiency. Every hour, take a 5-minute break to stretch or walk around, which encourages mitochondrial function by enhancing blood flow and oxygen supply.
- ***Eat a Mitochondria-Boosting Lunch:*** Opt for a nutrient-dense meal with sources of CoQ10 (like spinach or broccoli), B vitamins (from dark leafy

greens or seeds), and antioxidants. This can help protect mitochondria and support energy production through the afternoon.

- **_Limit Processed Carbohydrates and Sugars:_** These can create blood sugar spikes and crashes, taxing the mitochondria. Instead, incorporate complex carbs like quinoa, legumes, or sweet potatoes, which provide slow, sustained energy release.

3. Physical Activity for Mitochondrial Biogenesis

- **_Incorporate HIIT or Strength Training:_** High-Intensity Interval Training (HIIT) and resistance exercises stimulate mitochondrial biogenesis (the creation of new mitochondria) and improve mitochondrial efficiency. Aim for a few sessions per week to build both muscular and mitochondrial strength.

- ***Engage in Aerobic Exercise:*** Walking, cycling, swimming, or any form of aerobic exercise enhances the mitochondria's ability to produce ATP, the main energy molecule in cells. Try to fit in at least 30 minutes of moderate aerobic exercise most days for best results.

4. Afternoon Rejuvenation and Focus on Antioxidants

- ***Snack on Antioxidant-Rich Foods:*** To reduce mitochondrial oxidative stress, have a snack with antioxidant-rich foods like blueberries, dark chocolate (70% cocoa or more), or green tea, which provide polyphenols that protect mitochondria from free radical damage.

- ***Practice Mindfulness or Breathing Exercises:*** Stress can produce free radicals that damage mitochondria. Incorporate deep breathing, meditation, or mindfulness activities to keep stress levels low and maintain mitochondrial resilience.

5. Evening Wind-Down for Recovery and Repair

- **Light Dinner Focused on Protein and Healthy Fats:** Protein provides amino acids, which are essential for cellular repair, including in mitochondria. Healthy fats from foods like salmon, olive oil, or nuts support mitochondrial membranes and improve cellular energy production.

- **Turn Off Electronic Devices 1-2 Hours Before Bed:** Blue light exposure at night interferes with melatonin production, which can impair mitochondrial repair processes that happen during sleep. Instead, create a calming, device-free bedtime routine that promotes optimal sleep.

- **Supplement Smartly if Needed:** If advised by a healthcare provider, consider supplements that support mitochondrial health, such as magnesium, CoQ10, and B vitamins, which play key roles in cellular energy production and mitochondrial repair.

6. Prioritize Quality Sleep for Mitochondrial Restoration

- ***Aim for 7-9 Hours of Sleep:*** Mitochondria repair and regenerate during deep sleep stages, making quality sleep crucial for mitochondrial health. Maintain a consistent sleep schedule, aiming to go to bed and wake up at the same times each day.

- ***Reduce Stimulants Before Bed***: Avoid caffeine and heavy meals in the evening, which can disrupt sleep quality. Herbal teas with calming properties, like chamomile or peppermint, can promote restful sleep without overstimulating your body.

7. Weekly Detoxification Practices

- ***Try Intermittent Fasting (if appropriate):*** Intermittent fasting can stimulate autophagy, a process where cells remove damaged mitochondria, allowing new, efficient mitochondria to thrive. Popular approaches include the 16:8 method (fasting for 16 hours and eating within an 8-hour window) if it aligns with your health needs.

- ***Consider Sauna or Epsom Salt Baths:*** Heat exposure from a sauna can promote mitochondrial resilience, while Epsom salt baths offer magnesium, which relaxes muscles and supports mitochondrial function.

A holistic approach to mitochondrial health emphasizes regular movement, balanced meals, stress management, and sufficient sleep. By integrating these daily routines, you support the mitochondria in generating energy efficiently, reducing oxidative stress, and enabling your body to maintain energy and resilience for long-term health.

Boosting mitochondrial health through lifestyle practices can transform your overall energy levels, cognitive function, and resilience against stress.

Incorporating the right exercise, sleep, and stress management techniques can create a ripple effect that supports not just your mitochondria but your entire well-being. explore some key practices that can power up your cells and fuel you through your days.

Exercise for Mitochondrial Function

Exercise is one of the most effective ways to stimulate mitochondrial biogenesis, or the formation of new mitochondria. Our muscles and cells adapt to physical demands, and exercise, particularly the right kind, can encourage mitochondria to multiply and become more efficient at producing energy. But not all exercise impacts mitochondria the same way.

1. High-Intensity Interval Training (HIIT)

HIIT is a game-changer for mitochondrial health. This type of workout alternates between short bursts of intense activity and recovery periods. For instance, imagine sprinting at full speed for 20 seconds, followed by 40 seconds of walking to recover. These intervals push your cells to adapt to the energy demand, effectively signaling mitochondria to increase their efficiency and multiply.

When I started adding HIIT into my routine, I noticed a shift in my energy levels throughout the day. Just 20 minutes of HIIT, three times a week, was all it took to feel more awake and alert.

2. Aerobic Exercise for Endurance

Activities like brisk walking, swimming, and cycling promote oxygen flow and train your cells to use oxygen efficiently, supporting long-lasting energy production. Aerobic exercise gently stresses your mitochondria, making them more efficient over time, which means more endurance for you in both physical activities and day-to-day tasks.

3. Strength Training for Mitochondrial Density

Strength training, whether with weights or body resistance, has profound effects on mitochondrial density in muscle cells. When you work your muscles, it signals your body to build more mitochondria to support energy needs for those muscles. Weight training is particularly beneficial as it increases both muscle mass and mitochondrial health.

Key Tips for Exercise Routine

- ***Start small if you're new:*** Begin with 5–10 minutes of any movement and gradually increase intensity.
- ***Listen to your body:*** Mitochondria benefit from exercise, but overdoing it can cause more stress than good.
- ***Consistency over intensity:*** While intense workouts are beneficial, regular moderate activity is equally important. Aim to stay active every day, even if it's a short walk or light stretching.

Sleep and Stress Management Techniques

The Vital Role of Quality Sleep

Sleep is the body's time for repair, and this includes mitochondrial repair. Mitochondria work tirelessly during the day, and nighttime is when they restore, detoxify, and prepare to support you for the next day. Without adequate sleep, mitochondria can't properly repair themselves, leading to cellular fatigue and, over time, impacting your overall health.

Sleep Tips to Maximize Mitochondrial Restoration:

- **_Prioritize Consistency:_** Going to bed and waking up at the same time every day supports a natural circadian rhythm, which mitochondria rely on to repair themselves.

- ***Limit Blue Light Exposure Before Bed:*** Electronic screens emit blue light, which suppresses melatonin, the hormone needed for quality sleep. Try switching off devices an hour before bed, or use blue-light-blocking glasses.
- ***Create a Calming Routine:*** Gentle stretches, meditation, or even reading can signal your body that it's time to wind down. Personally, a nightly ritual of stretching and a warm cup of herbal tea helps me sleep deeply.

Managing Stress for Mitochondrial Health

Mitochondria are highly responsive to stress, and while small doses of stress (like exercise) are beneficial, chronic stress can damage these powerhouses. When we're under constant stress, mitochondria shift from energy production to "survival mode," which reduces their efficiency.

Techniques to Keep Stress in Check

- ***Mindful Breathing:*** Deep breathing exercises, like the 4-7-8 method (inhale for 4 seconds, hold for 7, and exhale for 8) activate the parasympathetic nervous system, calming the mind and protecting mitochondria from stress overload.

- ***Regular Meditation:*** Even five minutes of mindfulness or meditation each day can significantly reduce stress. Studies show that regular meditation increases resilience, which helps mitochondria stay in balance. Apps like Headspace or Calm can guide you through short meditations if you're new to the practice.

- ***Gratitude Practice:*** It may sound simple, but reflecting on things you're grateful for each day can shift your mindset. Positive thinking has been shown to reduce stress markers in the body, indirectly supporting mitochondrial health.

When I first began incorporating these lifestyle practices, I was surprised by the ripple effect they had on my energy and well-being. For example, prioritizing consistent sleep was one of the simplest yet most profound changes I made. By creating a calming nighttime routine, I started noticing improvements not only in my energy levels but also in my mood and mental clarity. The power of supporting mitochondrial health through small, intentional habits can make a huge difference.

By making simple but powerful changes in exercise, sleep, and stress management, you're giving your mitochondria the support they need to power you through life with vitality. Mitochondria respond to our daily routines and habits, so embracing these practices with intention can help you enjoy sustained energy, clearer thinking, and a greater sense of well-being.

Conclusion

The New Mitochondria Diet brings a fresh approach to achieving optimal health by nourishing the very core of our cellular energy system: the mitochondria.

Mitochondria, often called the "powerhouses" of the cell, are responsible for creating the energy that fuels every aspect of our lives—from physical vitality to mental clarity and resilience against stress and disease.

By focusing on specific nutrients, balanced eating patterns, and lifestyle adjustments that support mitochondrial health, this diet offers a pathway to enhanced energy, longevity, and overall wellness.

Throughout this book, we've explored how mitochondrial function can be profoundly influenced by what we eat and how we live. With a strong emphasis on antioxidant-rich foods, anti-inflammatory ingredients, and nutrients like CoQ10, magnesium, and omega-3s, the New Mitochondria Diet is designed to reduce oxidative stress and inflammation, which are major threats to mitochondrial health. Each recipe and meal plan has been carefully crafted to deliver the essential nutrients that help protect, repair, and even build new mitochondria, providing a sustainable source of energy and resilience.

But the benefits extend beyond nutrition. Supporting mitochondria involves a holistic approach that includes exercise, sleep, and stress management. Small, intentional lifestyle changes—like prioritizing sleep, incorporating restorative exercises, and practicing mindfulness—help create a balanced environment in which mitochondria thrive.

Whether you're just beginning your wellness journey or are looking to enhance an already healthy lifestyle, this diet is a resource for anyone interested in optimizing energy and promoting long-term vitality. Embracing the principles of the New Mitochondria Diet can empower you to live with more energy, sharper mental clarity, and greater resilience, supporting a fulfilling, vibrant life. Here's to nurturing your mitochondria and unlocking a new level of health and well-being!

www.ingramcontent.com/pod-product-compliance
Lightning Source LLC
Chambersburg PA
CBHW071220260726
48653CB00042B/1434